Nourish

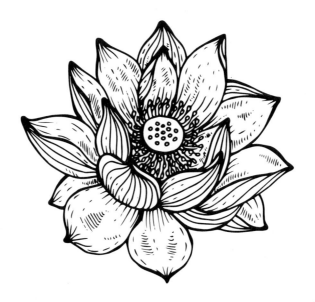

Stephanie Hrehirchuk

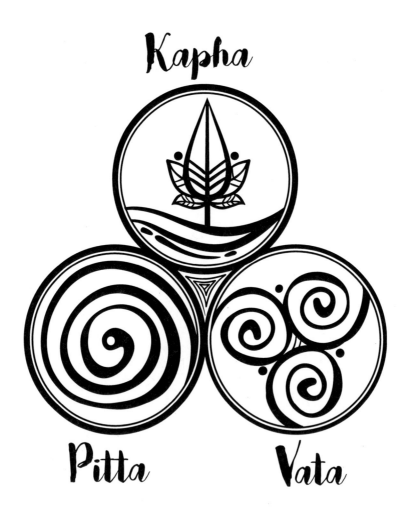

Nourish

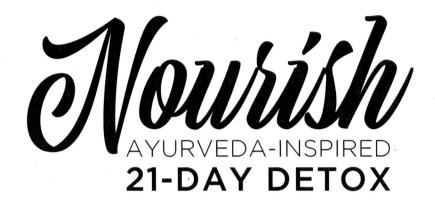

AYURVEDA-INSPIRED
21-DAY DETOX

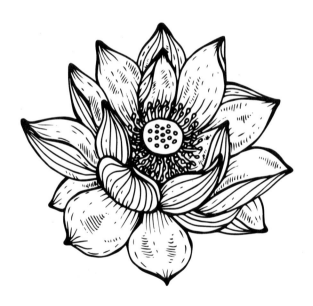

Stephanie Hrehirchuk

Nourish: Ayurveda-inspired 21-day Detox

Published by Anna's Angels Press

Copyright © 2017 Stephanie Hrehirchuk

Copy editor: Maraya Loza Koxahn

Cover image by Stephanie Hrehirchuk

Book design by Robyn Monkman

ISBN (Print) 978-0-9958839-5-6
ISBN (eBook) 978-0-9958839-4-9

Printed on recycled paper

The information presented here represents the views of the author as of the date of publication. This program is meant to inform, not diagnose or treat specific health conditions. It is not a substitute for professional medical advice, diagnosis and treatment. Always consult your doctor before beginning an exercise, wellness or nutrition plan.

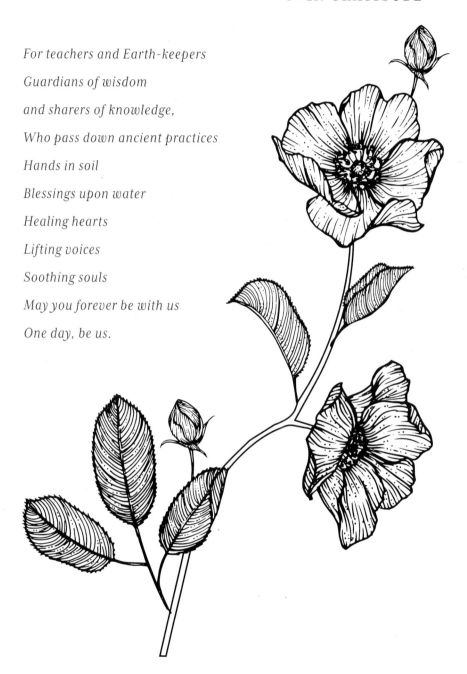

ℰ In gratitude

For teachers and Earth-keepers

Guardians of wisdom

and sharers of knowledge,

Who pass down ancient practices

Hands in soil

Blessings upon water

Healing hearts

Lifting voices

Soothing souls

May you forever be with us

One day, be us.

CONTENTS

My Story..11

Why Detox?...17

Your key to success....................................21

Emotional support......................................22

21-Day Detox...23

      Detox Prep..25

      Welcome to Week One...............................31

      Welcome to Week Two...............................37

      Welcome to Week Three.............................41

Next Steps...45

3-day Reset..47

DIY Self-care..49

Seasonal balance.......................................57

      Spring..58

      Summer..59

      Fall..63

      Winter..65

Also by Stephanie Hrehirchuk.................................71

Meet the Author..72

We need more than a detox that deals solely with diet. We need a detox that nourishes body, mind and spirit.

IN THIS PROGRAM, I combine the dietary wisdom of 15 years of experience working with fitness and nutrition clients, with self-care practices offered by Ayurveda: India's 5,000-year-old science of life.

You don't need to understand Ayurveda in order to benefit from the 21-day detox, although I believe you will enjoy the program so much, you will want to investigate Ayurveda further.

Through my years of working with clients in nutrition and wellness, I understand firsthand the importance of encouragement, support, enjoyable routines, and accountability.

I also know the power of community.

Which is why I welcome you to join the private Facebook group:

Nourish: Ayurveda-inspired 21-day detox

Another gift for you to help with your success: please download the free workbook at stephaniehrehirchuk.com

These additional resources will support you in getting the most from your program.

In the Facebook group, we move through the detoxes together, seasonally, though you are welcome to enjoy the program whenever it suits you.

If you are not on Facebook, (or even if you are), create your own 21-day detox group with friends and members of your community. Go through the program together and swap recipes, offer support and accountability to each other.

Speak only when your words are
more beautiful than the silence.
~ Arabic proverb

MY STORY

AN ATHLETE FROM the age of 12, I was a personal trainer by the age of 26. For 15 years, I created personal training programs for clients based on nutrition and exercise. Although effective in their purpose, diet and exercise only proved part of the puzzle.

I suffered a spinal injury at age 31 which eventually forced me from my passion and career as a personal trainer. My body had always complied brilliantly with my orders, until the day I could no longer walk; that day, my body started *giving* the orders

Thankfully, my bed-ridden days numbered only 33, and I was back on my feet. Although not completely functional, I fully expected to return to my life of exercise. My body had other plans. I managed to make it to my wedding, only weeks after I had returned to my feet, and delivered two beautiful children in the following years. I tried to live life as I saw fit, but my back always dictated the terms of my day.

What frustrated me the most was that I had lived a life that anyone would have considered the epitome of health. I did all the right things. How could I have ended up in such poor condition?

I found yoga, and by age 37, had a daily practice and offered classes in my home studio. Yoga poses easily replaced my lost weights and cardio routine, and I began to bend and move my body in exciting new ways. I thought I'd found my cure.

My body pushed back through buckling knees and back spasms. I may have picked up an extra puzzle piece but I still didn't have the whole picture.

On a trip to the local organic grocery store, I stumbled upon a lemon balm plant. I was fascinated by the green beauty with its fuzzy lemony leaves. I brought lemon balm home and my herbal love affair began.

Then the Ayurvedic Institute crossed my path. I was determined to study Marma therapy with Dr. Vasant Lad, the Institute's founder. The class was full. The only other available course that suited my schedule was a weekend in Ayurvedic Herbology. It seemed serendipitous, on the heals of my new-found plant passion, so I hopped a plane from Calgary to Albuquerque.

Grateful for Dr. Lad's wealth of sharing, yet overwhelmed with the vast number of herbal elixirs and recipes, I returned home and tucked my notebook away. The flights, however, had wreaked havoc on my back, and I was soon researching Ayurvedic treatments for herniated discs. I found a specific treatment and proceeded to search for anyone offering it in my city. I was certain the chances of finding someone were slim and none.

Synchronicity struck again; I found one local Ayurvedic practitioner and after several therapeutic sessions and many conversations, she offered to come to my home studio and talk about *panchakarma,* a traditional Ayurvedic detox program, with my clients. We paired her program with the yoga classes I offered.

I loved both facilitating and participating in the program, and began to make adjustments to the content based on my years of experience working with personal training clients, and the feedback from the program participants. After four years of facilitating seasonal detox programs, it was time to bring the program into book form, so that you can bring it into your home, health and life.

Through my 10 years of exploration and studies in complementary and alternative medicine, I was in constant pursuit of healing my body so I could get back to fitness. What I came to realize was that the very condition I was fighting to fix, not only spurred me on to explore alternative modalities and ancient practices, but also showed me how responsible my state of mind was for the state of my body, and how limited my thinking was in terms of health. Diet and exercise are certainly big pieces of a puzzle, and go a long way toward mental and emotional health, but not all the way.

My spine told me that I needed to restore balance in my body and mind. Ayurveda taught me how.

I find Ayurveda equally powerful and poetic, complex and comprehensive, and timeless and timely. I discovered that I have an opportunity to build a bridge between what we in the west have come to accept as good for our health and what those in the east have known for millennia as a path to balance.

Nourish is that bridge. Here, I offer the nutrition practices that I have found most beneficial for clients over the years, and added the self-care piece that is sorely lacking from our daily living. This program is designed to assist you in creating a daily wellness routine that is not only aimed at detoxification, but nourishment of body, mind and spirit.

My intention is to deliver a simple, elegant and effective program that inspires a deeper connection to your physical, mental and emotional self, and the way in which you nourish yourself and those around you every day.

May we be empowered in our choices

Supported in our practices

And encouraged in our endeavors.

May we be light in mood

Happy in heart

And easeful in body.

May we all be

Nourished.

"When we look at the lives of great creative souls, we find that they feel themselves to be hooked up to, guided, incarnated, or allied by a power that is beyond or deep within themselves."

~ Jean Houston

WHY DETOX?

Over the years, we accumulate residue from undigested and unprocessed material in the body. This residue effects not only the physical, but also the mental and emotional bodies. In Ayurveda, this accumulation is called *ama*, and Ayurveda cites ama as the root cause of disease. Seasonal detoxes are used to rid the body of ama and restore balance to the whole person.

Detox is designed to lighten the load on the body's organs and lessen inflammation before it contributes to chronic disease. This Ayurveda-inspired detox program is like hitting the reset button for the body, mind and spirit. It is designed to lighten the load on the emotions and mind, as well as the body. It is intended to assist you in creating a nourishing daily self-care ritual.

Everything is connected. Our diet affects our mental and emotional health. Our mental and emotional states affect our food choices and lifestyle habits. Our lifestyle habits affect our emotional state... and it goes on and on. Add to this circle: the seasons, those with whom we surround ourselves, and where we live. Our location affects the local food available, hours of sunlight and weather. The weather impacts what we eat and often drives our mood. Our family and community influence our diet, thoughts, emotions and practices.

Taking 21 days at the turn of each season, creates a window of awareness of all the forces that shape our lives and health, and allows us, through daily practice, to restore balance naturally.

We talk about self-care as if it were a luxury, something we treat ourselves to on special occasions: a massage on Mother's Day, a pedicure for summer, an annual weekend retreat. Self-care and self-love are two key missing pieces of our health puzzle. The Ayurveda-inspired practices included in this program are not only beneficial for detox, they are practices I encourage you to continue, in some form, as a daily deepening connection to self: through love and care.

Nourish is simple, easy to follow and a direct route to creating a daily self-care ceremony. It's about nourishing the body, inside and out.

When we nourish the self, we are better able to nourish our families, friends and communities. When our cup is full, we can more easily pour into another's.

Previous program participants have reported

- Weight Loss
- Improved Sleep
- Decreased Sense Of Stress
- Increased Energy
- Improved Eating Habits
- Improved Condition Of Skin
- Decreased Pain/Inflammation Of Joints
- Balanced Mood
- A Greater Feeling Of Well-Being
- Decreased Dependence On Sugar, Coffee And Caffeine Sources For Energy
- Benefits Of The Practices Long After Detox

*You should sit in meditation for 20
minutes every day - unless you're too
busy; then you should sit for an hour*

~ Old Zen adage

YOUR KEY TO SUCCESS

ᴔ ONE DAY AT A TIME

SHOW UP EACH day. Perform the practices for that day. Let go of any planned outcome, and be open to what's possible.

The program is designed in four segments, each lasting one week. You will start with a prep week and then be guided through the 21-day program, one week at a time. Move through each segment in order.

Words such as *diet* and *detox* trigger resistance, restriction and discomfort. Let's take the charge out of those words by replacing them with one that invokes wellbeing: *Nourish*.

Think less of it as what you cannot have to eat and
more from the perspective of what nourishing foods
you will include.

Once you have added all the nourishing parts of your food practice, you may discover there is little room, or interest, in less-nourishing food choices.

Although traditional detox is very much about the food, if the food part is creating antagonistic energy for you, please focus on the self-care practices and allow the foods, whatever foods you enjoy, to be nourishing.

There's no counting calories, or measuring portions or waistlines. We are returning to our nutrition intuition and deepening our relationship with food.

Relax and rediscover your innate ability to nourish your body, mind and spirit.

❧ EMOTIONAL SUPPORT

During the 21-day detox, you will **not** go hungry. You will be well-nourished. This does not mean that you won't still come face to face with the expression of stuffed emotions as they leave the body. Like guests at a party, you will discover who leaves graciously and who does not.

Emotions arise and often we feed them. This creates a pattern of supplication through substance, in this case: food. The practice of daily journaling will help you to understand more about yourself and your habits: why you do what you do, eat what and when you eat, and how you feed your body, mind and emotions.

Lama Tsultrim Allione authored a powerful book entitled *Feeding Your Demons*. I highly recommend it. Enhancing awareness of how you move through your day, particularly feeding your thoughts and deep-seated emotions, is one of the key facets of *Nourish*. Don't try to avoid your emotions. Try to meet them, see them, and breathe with them.

I recommend downloading the accompanying workbook found at stephaniehrehirchuk.com and using it to further facilitate your process during the program.

WELCOME TO YOUR

Ayurveda-inspired

21-DAY DETOX.

> *"There is not one life that doesn't add tremendous value to the whole. Somewhere inside of us we know this to be true; we hear the call to head in the direction of this bigger life."*
> *~ Debbie Ford*

DETOX PREP

The theme for this week is food preparation: getting ready for your detox.

❧ CLEAN OUT THE CUPBOARDS.

THIS IS THE week to use up, donate to the food bank, store away for later, or eliminate any processed and refined foods. Clean out the pantry and the fridge of foods that may pull you off track, and make room for fresh new fixings.

Gluten is out – pasta, bread, white and wheat flours, packaged cereals, buns, cookies, cakes, pizza crusts... you get the picture. Eliminate all processed foods and flours, including gluten-free baked goods.

Drop the sugar – chocolates, candies, confections and baking, ice cream, sweets. A quality honey or maple syrup, along with dates and fruit, will be your sweet allies during the detox.

Reduce dairy and meat – hard cheeses, milk, sour cream, ice cream, processed meats like sandwich meats, pre-seasoned or smoked meats are out.

Susan had no trouble omitting meat from her meals during the program. Other participants found that including a small amount of quality chicken or fish 2-3 times per week helped stabilize blood sugar and kept them from seeking sweets and snacks. Nuts, greens, chia seeds, cinnamon, and healthy fats like coconut oil, nut butters or avocado, are additional ways to assist with regulating blood sugar and keeping cravings at bay.

Don't stress about omitting foods. You won't go hungry. The idea is to get temptation out of the house and inflammation out of the body.

If this is your first detox, start with the removal of gluten, dairy and refined sugar. If this is not your first detox, or if your regular diet doesn't include these foods, use the 21 days to also remove eggs, corn, soy, and processed oils such as canola oil.

☙ ADVISE THE OTHER MEMBERS OF YOUR HOUSEHOLD ABOUT THE PLAN AND ENLIST THEIR SUPPORT.

IF YOU CAN enjoy the 21 days with your family, the process becomes even sweeter. If not, enlist a friend or two and be each other's accountability buddy. Of course, this is also where the Facebook group comes in handy. Share recipes, swap meal plans, and report your progress regularly.

My husband did not participate directly in my first detox. I advised him of my plan and asked him to indulge in the foods I was eliminating while he was at work during the day, and not to bring chips, sweets, treats and take-out food home.

In her first detox, Lisa found it easy to prepare a batch of kitcharee (ayurvedic dish of veggies and rice), or soup for herself to reheat for dinner while she prepared family favorites for the rest of her brood.

If you think you may succumb to temptation, don't have it on hand at all.

℅ IDENTIFY ANY WITCHING HOURS AND PUT A PLAN IN MOTION.

IF THERE IS a certain time of day that finds you poking around the pantry for sweet or salty, then crashing on the couch to indulge in front of the TV, or surf the world wide webs, commit to fill your witching hours with a walk outside. Or join a yoga or other movement or meditation class with a friend, read a book or take an art class.

℅ MAKE YOUR MEAL PLAN AND GROCERY LIST FOR WEEK ONE.

WHAT FOODS DO you enjoy? How can you modify your favorite meals? Experiment with new recipes or get inspiration from the Facebook group. Remember, you have this prep time to make a plan for week one.

Cindy found a delicious recipe for lentil shepherd's pie. Kirsten made a large batch of veggie soup and froze it for the coming weeks.

The prep that you do now makes the coming weeks easier. Start jotting down your ideas this week and whip up whatever inspires you to have on hand in order to keep life simple and nourishing.

- rice

- yams

- sweet potatoes

- potatoes

- chia seeds or a seedy porridge mix to eat hot or cold (buckwheat, hemp hearts, chia seeds, nuts and other seeds)

- veggies to eat fresh: carrot sticks, celery, peppers, cucumbers

- and ones for steaming, roasting or sautéing: broccoli, cauliflower, carrots, peppers, onion, garlic, bok choy, swiss chard, eggplant

- fruits such as apples, oranges, watermelon, berries, etc.

- **Fresh ginger** is nice to have on hand, grated into tea, water, or your favorite dishes, ginger stokes the digestive fire (*agni*).

- Make a batch of **baba ganouj** for a quick lunch with carrot and celery sticks or seedy crackers. Toss with your salad greens as a dressing.

- Create a **snack mix** for times when you may crave something sweet: pumpkin and sunflower seeds, raisins, cranberries, figs or dates to sweeten. Watch out for super salty pre-mixes or sweetened and sulphured dried fruit. Better to blend up your own.

- Make a big batch of **applesauce/cider** to enjoy hot or cold.

If you are a coffee-drinker, this is the week to begin a gradual decrease of your daily dose of joe. Likewise, with the evening glass of red or white, or happy hour beverage of choice. Begin to wean yourself of these habitual go-to's for energy or relaxation.

Lisa replaced her afternoon cup of coffee with a cup of tea and began reducing her morning cup of coffee to ¾, then ½, then ¼. She enjoyed a cup of guyusa tea in the morning to help move her from coffee.

Take a look at your own recipe repertoire and see where you can breathe new life into your meals.

Discover new recipes online.
Find an Ayurvedic cookbook or recipe site.

Don't eat past 6:30 p.m. and avoid snacking in the evening. This, alone, is a practice in food and self awareness. Perhaps an evening cup of herbal tea? Or an organic apple? Don't struggle. Find a nourishing solution.

Tanya substituted her regular heavy, sugary, evening snack with a small bowl of air-popped popcorn topped with a bit of coconut oil and sea salt.

Keep it simple. Plan your week's meals with similar ingredients for economy of use.

Use leftover rice from dinner for tomorrow's rice pudding, chicken and rice soup, or add greens, a few beans and fresh salsa for a Mexican rice salad.

Stir leftover lemon-roasted kale potatoes into baba ganouj for a quick and delicious potato salad lunch. Top with fresh greens.

A BIG piece of the puzzle is food. No matter how wonderful or powerful the other practices are, I always hear "I don't know what to eat!"

Changing our dietary habits should not feel distressing. We wish to facilitate a loving relationship with food, not a contentious one. Over the years that I have run this program, I found the one area where clients couldn't get enough support is always tied up in food.

Detox tip: if it **has** ingredients, don't eat it. If it **is** an ingredient, eat it. And combine it with other ingredients to create a nourishing, whole foods meal.

The most effective way for me to respond to this piece of the puzzle, is to offer a more engaging and dynamic format for food. Join the private Facebook group where recipes are shared in accordance with the seasons.

This forum not only provides fresh food inspiration, but it also offers community, support and accountability. I encourage you to join. Look for Nourish: Ayurveda-inspired 21-day Detox **on Facebook.**

Happy prep!

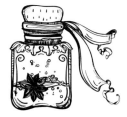

> *"The attitude of gratitude is
> the highest yoga."*
> ~ *Yogi Bhajan*

WELCOME TO WEEK ONE

This week is all about breath, water and gratitude. These three simple practices are the foundation for good health.

This week we create a morning and evening practice.

❦ MORNING

HOT WATER

(Not too hot. We don't want to burn the sensitive tissues of the mouth or throat).

DRINK ½ - 1 cup of heated water first thing in the morning. Water is one of the most receptive and malleable medicines. Water will take on the qualities of what surrounds it or is immersed in it. You may wish to infuse your water with a morning blessing or sweet word, or even chant or sing to your water before drinking. This practice alone, done each day, is very beneficial to health.

Chant *Om Namah Shivaya* seven times over your water.

This loving invocation of Lord Shiva contains the sounds which represent all five of the elements. Feel these elements come into balance within you as you sip your water.

GRATITUDE

JOURNAL THREE THINGS specific to each day, for which you are grateful. Avoid the generality of writing family, friends, home, etc. Be specific. Today, I am grateful for the bus arriving on time. I am grateful for my friend, Tammy, who took the time to listen to me share my excitement about my detox program. I am grateful for the quiet beauty of the flowering plum in my front yard. Journal three gifts of gratitude each night.

FOOTSIES

RUB THE SOLES of your feet with oil. You can use coconut oil, sweet almond, sesame, or even olive oil. You can infuse your oil with spices like clove or ginger, herbs such as lemon balm or basil, or add essential oils like lavender, sandalwood or rose geranium. Start with the left foot and massage the ball of the foot, under your toes, your instep and anywhere that feels good. Avoid the heels if you are concerned about oil on your sheets. Or use only a small amount of oil, or wear socks if that is comfortable.

Our feet are a goldmine of reflexology points and rubbing them with oil each night helps to stimulate these points and assists in the detoxification process.

Nadi Shodhana

NADI SHODHANA, OR ALTERNATE nostril breathing, is a powerful practice in itself. If I could recommend only one practice, it would be this one.

Perform 10-20 rounds of alternate nostril breathing before sleep.

Sitting comfortably on your bed, or meditation cushion if that is your practice, rest your pointer and middle finger against the forehead, between the eyebrows. Block right nostril with the thumb. Inhale through left nostril, block left nostril with fourth finger, release thumb and exhale through right nostril. Inhale through the right nostril, close with thumb, open left nostril and exhale. Inhale left, switch fingers, exhale right. Inhale right, switch fingers, exhale left.

Slow and deepen the breath as you relax the body. Spine is straight, chin tucked slightly, release tension in the shoulders and the belly. Close the eyes. Continue slowing and deepening the breath as you continue for 10-20 cycles of alternate nostril breathing. Allow the body to relax as the breath slows and the mind along with it.

You may wish to add the mantra *So Hum* (I am that), silently repeating Sooooooooooooooooo on the inhale and Hummmmmmmmmm on the exhale to keep the mind focused and promote clarity and connection between breath, body and mind. Work toward 11 minutes of practice, then rest your hands in your lap and allow your breath to return to both nostrils before slipping between the sheets for sweet slumber.

If your nasal passages feel blocked, you may wish to blow your nose before practice. Breathe calmly and steadily, exercising patience and encouraging ease with each breath. If your mind wanders, gently bring it back to the breath and So Hum.

However long you have to commit to this practice, alternate nostril breathing is one of the most beneficial practices you can add to your daily routine. Breathing practice works to open the *nadis*, or channels, of the body and strengthens the body, mind and spirit connection. If you have a yoga practice, please continue during the detox, if suitable. If you have yet to explore yoga, let the *pranayama*, or breathing practice, in this program be your yoga.

ℰ DETOX DRINK

A detoxifying Ayurvedic infusion to sip through the day:

- Boil water in the kettle
- Steep the following for 20-30 minutes in one cup hot water:
- 1 tbsp. blend of cumin seeds, fennel seeds and coriander seeds. Strain.
- Pour into a 1 litre bottle and top with fresh water to fill.
- Sip between meals, stopping by dinner.

Cumin is used to aid digestion, balance hypoglycemia, and is also a source of magnesium – which aids calcium absorption. Coriander is used to ease stomach upset, intestinal gas, and joint pain, as well as lower blood sugar levels and improve skin issues. It is also a diuretic. Fennel is used for irritable bowl, heartburn, bloating, upper respiratory issues, cough and backache. Together they ease the process of detoxification.

AWARENESS EXERCISE:

HOW ARE YOU taking your meals? Do you eat on the run? Over the kitchen sink? In the car? In front of the TV or computer? Are you sitting comfortably? Relaxed? Do you savor your food? Chew well? Are you in good company when you eat?

Your mental and emotional states, as well as physical, contribute to either good or poor digestion. Poor digestion contributes to ama. Always eat while sitting comfortably. Enjoy your food. Enjoy your company: whether family, friends or self. Take three deep breaths before you eat. Draw forth a sense of gratitude for the abundance of nourishment available to you. Relax the shoulders and the belly. Do not stuff yourself; 75-80% full is sufficient.

It is not about right or wrong, good or bad. It's no use inviting shame, blame or guilt to dinner. It's simply awareness. Noticing the current conditions and considering something different, something Nourishing.

---

*"Because we cannot scrub our inner body
we need to learn a few skills to help
cleanse our tissues, organs, and mind.
This is the art of Ayurveda."*

~ Sebastian Pole

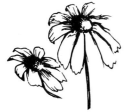

WELCOME TO WEEK TWO

This week we add two practices and a salt bath.

♌ DRY BRUSHING

PERFORM DRY BRUSHING before your morning shower or evening bath. You can generally purchase a dry brush at your local health food store or pharmacy. It's like a shower brush that you don't use with water. Dry brushing is used for exfoliation of the skin as well as stimulation of the lymphatic system.

Dry brush the entire body (toe to torso), avoiding the delicate skin on the face, breasts and neck.

Start brushing at the feet and move upward, in circular motion around the joints (ankles, knees, hips, shoulders, elbows, wrists) and straight strokes on the long bones (shins, thighs, arms), drawing the strokes repeatedly up the body toward the torso.

Then move to oil massage.

ꙮ *Abhyanga* (Self-massage)

ABHYANGA IS DAILY self massage with medicated oils. It is used to assist the body in removing toxins as well as absorbing the nutrients from the oil and herbs.

It is best to perform abhyanga before getting into the bath or shower (careful not to oil the soles of the feet so you don't slip). Use a quality oil (almond, sesame, coconut, or olive). You may wish to infuse your oil with herbs, add essential oils or simply apply plain.

You will find some delicious DIY recipes for body-care starting on page 49.

You may wish to place your bottle of oil into a container of hot water to warm the oil before you apply.

Again, use straight strokes on the long bones and circular motion on the joints, toward the torso. Avoid areas of injured, swollen or damaged skin. Ayurveda does not advise practicing abhyanga when pregnant, menstruating or during times of illness, though elements of gentle self-massage may be beneficial during these times. Always consult your healthcare practitioner.

Rub the belly in a circular motion, moving hands up the right side, across the top and down the left side, across the bottom and repeat. Rub the kidney area or have a partner rub oil along the spine and back. It is also nice to massage oil into the scalp. You will need to apply shampoo before water when you shower in order to remove the oil effectively.

The whole body massage should take only 5-15 minutes, but take as long as you like. You may also wish to book an appointment for an abhyanga massage by trained practitioners at an Ayurvedic spa.

Dry brushing and abhyanga may be done each morning before your shower, or, if you find it more convenient, in the evening before your bath. Whether you prefer to shower or bathe, set aside the time for three salt baths this week.

Run the bath while you preform dry brushing. When done, place a towel on the edge of the bathtub or a stool and enjoy your self-massage. Then add your salt to the water before stepping into the bath (ensure bottoms of feet have not been oiled).

Investigate the best salt for you: Himalayan salt, Dead Sea salt, epsom salts, baking soda or a combination. Start with 1 cup of salts and work up to 2 cups by the end of this week. Soak for 15-20 minutes then towel dry. The oil should have absorbed nicely into the skin with no need to reapply.

If you bathe before bed, oil the soles of the feet after your bath, complete your alternate nostril breathing and then off to sleep you go.

By now, you should have a morning practice of hot water and an evening practice of breathing. Add your dry brushing and self-massage to either time and create space for your salt baths. This need not take long. Again, take all the time you need. **Your number one priority this week is your own self-care.**

Nourish, massage, breathe, stretch your body and get plenty of water and rest.

"The great thing about Ayurveda is that its treatments always yield side benefits, not side effects."

~ Shubhra Krishan

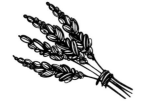

WELCOME TO WEEK THREE

This week we lose the electronics.

Less screen time = more ME time. More time to do your practices.

ᘓ DIGITAL DETOX

IT IS IMPORTANT to set the tone at the start of the day and before bed. These two times are key windows to wellbeing.

This week, power off your devices two hours before bed, but no later than 8:30 p.m. **And commit to not powering up again until two hours after you awake.** If your cell phone is your only phone, instead of powering it off, put it away somewhere where it is available in case of emergency, but not available for texting, chatting, surfing or gaming.

Use your morning time for self-care, breakfast, getting kids to school or yourself to the office, and setting a tone for your day.

MAKE IT A DAILY JOURNAL EXERCISE:
"Today I am..."

- ✺ grateful
- ✺ energized
- ✺ calm
- ✺ productive
- ✺ creative
- ✺ peaceful
- ✺ focused

A morning practice I enjoy is writing down the three most important things I need to do that day and focus on their completion. This may be three items related to work, or often it's two work items and a long walk in nature or a self-care practice, if I haven't made the time recently.

The practice is in taking the time to check in to what's important to me this day, before the energy and needs of family, friends, clients, coworkers or social media get involved, and making those three items a priority.

No more than three, so choose wisely. Perhaps it's only one. Some days it is sending out a thank you card or prepping the evening's dinner in advance. The quiet, contemplative space of morning practice provides clarity as to my heart's joyful desires and my soul's gentle nudging.

I love waking early. It can take some getting used to, but the practice of early rising affords me time to nourish myself, so that I can nourish my family in turn. The early, quiet hours are, indeed, some of the most magical hours of the day. Use your morning for hot water practice, dry brushing and self-massage, a morning walk, meditation, yoga or writing.

Rather than allow your emails or newsfeed to set the tone for your day, spend time with yourself and family and choose the tone you intend.

Again, in the evening, don't allow your social media, TV programs, work emails, or texts from friends to end your day. **Power off at least two hours before bed**. Spend this time cleaning up from your day and preparing for the next day.

Tend to your family and self, do your abhyanga and salt bath, alternate nostril breathing and complete your day with a note of gratitude in your journal. You may choose to extend the gratitude practice to family members, with each member sharing three things for which they are grateful, before turning in for the night.

ॐ

Get outside! Whether you meditate on the front step before sunrise or enjoy a noon or post-work walk, get outdoors and soak up nature. **Breathe deep. Release tension. Listen.** Relax and open to the nurturing, supportive energy of Mother Nature.

Rather than turn on the TV in the evening, or surf social media – grab your dog, friend, neighbor, husband, children or your lovely self and get outdoors. Breathe as if all the life force you could ever need is found in nature. And smile. Inhale peace, contentment, ease; exhale harmony, happiness and joy. Share your love and care with the world. Don't underestimate the healing power of nature.

࿐THIS WEEK, BRING ALL YOUR PRACTICES TOGETHER.

- Deepen your experience and commitment for the next seven days.
- Morning practice of hot water.
- Daily dry brushing/ abhyanga/salt bath.
- Evening foot rubs/alternate nostril breathing/ journaling.
- Keep eating vibrant, nourishing foods.

"Keep up and you'll be kept up."

~ Yogi Bhajan

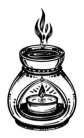

NEXT STEPS

CONTINUE WITH PRACTICES that nourish you: alternate nostril breathing in the evening, hot water in the morning, oil massage once or twice a week (even daily if you like), and gratitude journaling. Keep eating nourishing foods.

Slowly and gradually reintroduce gluten, dairy and sugar, if you choose. Consider keeping these ingredients at a minimum.

Relax into the foods and flavors of the season. Local and organic are always great choices. Return to the 21-day detox three weeks before the start of the next season, or as you feel guided.

Each time you return to the program, your recipe repertoire expands, your connections within the private Facebook group deepen, as does the connection to your sense of well-being.

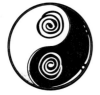

*"Good-humored patience is
necessary with mischievous
children and your own mind."*

~ Jack Kornfield

3-DAY RESET

CREATIVE PROJECTS ARE on the rise – spilling out onto scrap pieces of paper around the house – and I notice the portion of chocolate-covered pretzels has steadily increased while yoga has decreased as my source of fuel.

Rather than plow through and set myself up for a full detox, I choose a 3-day reset to restore balance in my body, my work, my creativity, and my sanity.

&ampersand; THERE ARE FIVE PARTS TO MY 3-DAY RESET:

1. Sweat and stretch. I replace my home yoga practice with a trip to a yoga studio for a warm flow class, peer support and a deeply detoxifying hour of sweating, breathing, and stretching. I take one litre of mountain spring water with me, complete with added flower essences to support my practice. If you prefer, grab a cycling class or Zumba, dance class or mall walking. Show up all three days for class.

2. Liquid nourishment. I hit the grocery store pre 3-day reset and grab beets, carrots, chard or greens of choice, and apples. Ginger, too, if you like. I found fresh pea shoots this time – why not? I juice enough vegetables for two cups of juice and add two cups of mountain spring water, put the blend in a pitcher in the fridge and drink throughout the day. Or, you may prefer a warm version of liquid nourishment: clove, ginger and cinnamon-spiced apple cider or strong chai tea. Your morning cup of ginger and lemon water will also serve nicely.

3. Eat clean. I keep dairy, gluten, and sugar at bay for the 3-day stay at Reset-ville. I enjoy rice, veggies and chicken or fish. I snack on spiced nuts and goji berries, and warm my belly with chai porridge of chia seeds, hemp hearts, apples, coconut oil, ginger, cardamom and cinnamon.

4. Get salty. A daily detox bath with Himalayan salts, Dead Sea salts, or herbal salt blend of choice, provides nourishing hydrotherapy. Add essential oils of mint and lavender or deeply-relaxing neroli. Grapefruit is energizing and sweet orange provides a lift. Petitgrain is purifying.

5. Play footsies. Self-massage helps with the reset and connects you to your body. Enjoy dry brushing and self-massage every day before your salt bath. Once out of the tub, pay particular attention to your feet. Give yourself a reflexology treatment as you rub rich cocoa butter or oil into your tender tootsies. Better yet, if you have a willing companion, exchange foot rubs with one another. Don't forget the kids. Rubbing your little ones' little piggies is a nourishing way to send them off to dreamtime.

If your plate is full and there is more to do on the horizon, don't wait for a 21-day break to get a handle on your health. Try a 3-day reset and restore balance naturally.

"Beauty is not in the face;
beauty is a light in the heart."
~ Kahlil Gibran

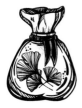

DIY SELF-CARE

CRAFTING YOUR OWN herbal oils is a nourishing ritual. A do-it-yourself day of kitchen chemistry can yield a season's worth of food for the senses.

VANILLA BEAN-INFUSED BALM
Infusing the whole vanilla bean gives this balm a natural, full aroma.

Step 1. Start by infusing your oil of choice with vanilla beans. Split the bean and scrape the *caviar* into the jar, then drop the bean in as well. Two to three beans per 500 mls will produce a divine aroma.

Sweet almond, coconut and light vegetable oils work best as a carrier. The lighter the aroma of the oil, the cleaner the vanilla scent will be.

Choose the best quality oil as this is what your body's largest organ, your skin, will be drinking in.

Fill the jar to the top with oil, no room for air, and cap tightly. Allow to infuse for 30 days in a warm windowsill or, if pressed for time, use a hot water bath to extract the essence.

This produces a delicious smelling oil that can be applied directly onto the skin as a luxurious body oil or poured into the bath for a relaxing soak.

Step 2. Pour the vanilla bean-infused oil into the top of a double boiler and add a quality beeswax. I'm really not one to measure, however, the last batch I made used about 150 ml of infused oil and 30 ml of beeswax, a couple tablespoons, perhaps.

Heat the mixture gently until the beeswax melts into the oil. Test the consistency by removing the spoon with a little of the mixture on it. It will cool quickly and give you an indication of how hard it will be once set.

If it is softer than you'd like, add more beeswax and continue to heat until melted. If it is too hard, add more infused oil and repeat the test until you reach the consistency you desire.

Remove the mixture from heat, making sure absolutely no water from the double boiler gets into your blend. Add a splash of vitamin E if you have it, for a natural preservative and pour the mixture into your clean, dry containers. When cooled, cap them and they are ready to go.

A yummy treat for chapped lips, dry skin, cracked heels or a soft, natural perfume for wrists and neck.

Variations

1. Add a little sweet orange essential oil to create a scent that will make everyone feel like a kid again.

2. The addition of essential oil of lavender produces a most relaxing blend. Soothing to the skin and the senses.

(If adding essential oils, choose therapeutic grade oils. Shake your creations well in order to disperse the oils evenly before use.)

You now have two delicious creations for the skin: your sensual vanilla bean-infused body oil and the beautiful vanilla-infused bee balm.

CHAI SPICE BALM

One of my favorite balms for fall.

Individually infuse organic cinnamon, cardamom, ginger, clove and Madagascar vanilla beans in sweet almond oil or carrier oil of choice, blend together and add beeswax.

A warming lip balm, hydrating hand and cuticle balm or exotic, spicy natural perfume.

Spices can easily be infused together to simplify the process.

Separate infusions allow you to make further creations like **cinnamon** oil and cocoa butter for a Valentine's foot rub. Or use the **clove** oil for a sore muscle and joint rub.

Infused in food grade organic carrier oils such as olive or sesame, clove oil can be used as a mouthwash or to soothe toothaches.

Cardamom provides an aromatic base for natural perfume. Add a small amount of essential oils of sandalwood and bergamot for a warm citrus blend or try neroli or rosewood. Blend cardamom with the vanilla infusion for a simple, exotic scent.

A hint of **lavender** essential oil added to the vanilla infusion creates a calm and relaxing blend. Vanilla beans infuse easily, imparting a full scent with a few beans.

Follow the steps for vanilla infused oil and balm. The balm recipe works for the chai spice blend as well. Many spices require more active methods of infusion than herbs. Use a heat bath or grind the spices to assist with a deep, rich scent.

In India, the origin of chai, unique family recipes are handed down through generations. Explore your spice rack for your signature chai blend.

Warm your skin, senses and soul this autumn with chai spice.

JASMINE GREEN TEA-INFUSED BODY BUTTER

This luxurious and pure body butter uses herb-infused oil to deliver the intelligence of the plant. Infuse any of your favorite herbs or aromatic teas for the beneficial properties of the phytonutrients.

Herb-infused oil

- Place herbs in a clean, dry jar, about ⅔ full.
- Add oil, stirring to release any bubbles and fill to the top, capping the jar.
- Infuse in a warm windowsill for 30 days or more and strain.
- Or add herbs to oil in a double boiler or water bath and gently heat for 30-60 minutes, strain and continue with the body butter.

You can skip the steps above by simply using a good quality oil like sweet almond, sesame or sunflower instead of an infused oil. The lighter the scent of the base oil, the more fragrant the scent of the infused oil.

This kitchen chemistry DIY is a one-dish, simple method for an indulgent and natural treat for your skin and senses.

Body butter

- Melt approximately **1½ cups of shea butter** in a double boiler over low heat.
- Once all the shea butter has melted, remove from heat and

add about ¾ **cup jasmine green tea-infused, other herb-infused or pure oil** and stir.

- Allow this mixture to cool but not completely set. I place mine in the deep freezer (or, if in the winter, I place it out in the snow for a little snow prana for about 15 minutes or until it just starts to set and then pull it out).

- Add approximately **1 tsp. of vitamin E**, if you have it, and **10 - 15 mls of essential oils**, depending upon the strength of the scent of the oil and how fragrant you would like your butter.

- Whip until smooth and creamy.

Fair trade shea butter is made from the pit of a fruit that grows wild in West Africa. Its production supports African women and their communities.

The making of shea butter is exclusively a female activity. The butter has been used for centuries to moisturize the skin and protect it from heat, wind and salt water.

Shea promotes soft, silky-smooth, hydrated skin.

Jasmine is adored for her aphrodisiac qualities and exotic fragrance.

Other body butter candidates include: mint, lavender, lemon balm, chai tea, rosemary, sweet orange, neroli, rose, vanilla...the possibilities are endless.

Spoon into clean dry containers and enjoy. Ideal for hands, heels, elbows and whatever other parts of the body need moisture. Always keep essential oils away from the eyes.

NATURAL MOUTHWASH: A FLAVORFUL PRACTICE
Simple, easy and most likely all ingredients are already in your pantry.

Many traditions have used various vegetable oils as mouthwash. In Ayurveda, sesame oil is used. A small amount is all that is needed to swish around vigorously in the mouth. The longer you swish, the more the oil mixes with saliva, drawing bacteria and toxins from the mouth to be spit out and rinsed away down the drain.

Rinse the mouth with fresh water a couple times, brush and you're good to go. Rinse the sink with hot water.

My preferred mouthwash involves a handful of dried clove buds added to my bottle of sesame oil. For a milder rinse, use the whole buds intact. Crush the buds for a more intense mouthwash.

Other spices to try include:

- Cinnamon
- Cardamom
- Ginger
- Vanilla pods
- Licorice root

Many of these act as disinfectants as they have antibacterial and antimicrobial properties and are also used in aiding issues of the mouth and gums.

You are essentially making an oil infusion. Pick your favorite or make a blend: chai mouthwash! Remember, each day your infusion will intensify, so start out mild and by the end of the bottle you could have quite the potent rinse.

A small bottle will last a long time as you need only a tablespoon per use. If the bottom of the bottle is too strong, add more oil. If sesame is not on hand or your oil of choice, try olive or coconut. Coconut oil is solid at room temperature. You can heat it gently to infuse the herbs. It will set again once cool. The heat in your mouth will melt it when you swish. Clove-infused coconut oil also makes a great toothpaste.

Choose a quality oil, as well as spices, preferably organic or pesticide-free.

In Ayurveda, bad breath is often a sign of an improper diet. If you experience chronic bad breath, consider making a few dietary adjustments to restore balance to your digestive system. In the meantime, nourish your teeth and gums with your own spicy mouthwash.

ORGANIC LAVENDER BUD-INFUSED OIL

- Fill a clean, dry glass jar ⅔ full of dried lavender buds.

- Top with oil of choice, stir to remove any trapped air bubbles and fill the jar completely with oil.

- Cap tightly and shake, turn, sing to or dance with your beautiful infusion daily for up to 30 days.

- Alternatively, place your jar in a warm water bath and gently heat while stirring or lightly macerating the buds with a utensil or pestle for 20-40 minutes to provide same-day herbal oil.

- Strain the herbs and pour the oil into a clean, dry container.

- Add a bit of vitamin E if you have it or rosemary oil or extract for a preservative and a nice blend.

- Store in a cool, dry place.

- Massage directly onto skin, add a couple tbsps. to a warm bath or add to melted beeswax for a soothing skin balm.

- Ideal for mild sunburns, scrapes, scratches, inflamed or reactive skin, or for simply relaxing.

The lavender buds that you strained: add to your bath for a decadent home spa treatment. Or to Dead Sea or Himalayan salts for a body scrub. Add more oil as needed. So many self care ideas from one simple infusion.

Pour love into your kitchen creations. And let that love pour back onto your body through your nourishing self-care practices.

Always keep essential oils out of the reach of children. Consult your healthcare practitioner before use if pregnant. Dilute essential oils before applying to skin. Essential oils are powerful. A little goes a long way.

"A society grows great when old men plant trees whose shade they know they shall never sit in."

~ Greek Proverb

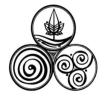

SEASONAL BALANCE

AYURVEDA LOOKS TO Nature in order to understand our own nature: the five elements – earth, water, fire, air and space – that exist within each one of us in different quantities and combinations.

Ayurveda recognizes these elements through the three *doshas*: **Vata** (Air & Space), **Pitta** (Fire & Water) and **Kapha** (Earth & Water). While all three doshas are present in each of us, we likely have one or two dominant dosha(s) that provide our unique physical, mental and emotional characteristics. When there is ama in the body, excess doshas may stick to this ama and create dis-ease. We use diet, self-care and lifestyle practices to pacify the excess dosha(s), and clear ama from the body.

While we manage our individual nature, or constitution, there are also the seasons to be considered. Each season expresses a particular combination of doshas and can contribute to excess qualities of those doshas, pulling us off balance, (or nudging us toward balance, depending upon your unique constitution), as the seasons change. A predominantly pitta person may struggle with the heat of summer yet find the cooling season of fall naturally nourishing.

As the seasons change, it is important to modify our diet in order to maintain balance. The salads that kept you cool in the heat of summer may not serve you as well in the midst of winter. Ayurveda shines a light on maintaining harmony year-round.

୫ SPRING

'TIS THE SEASON of spring cleaning. Spring energies spur us into action: cleaning out the closets; cleaning out the cupboards; and cleaning out the pipes. This is a prime season to detox.

Early spring is still kapha season (water and earth – heavy and wet). But as the frost comes out of the ground, kapha also begins to emerge from the body: mucous, congestion, runny nose. In Ayurveda, like increases like: if we add more wet, cold, heavy and oily onto this season, we will likely experience more mucous, congestion, oily skin, lethargy and dullness. The biggie here is excess.

Kapha craves excess sugar, sleep, bread, and fried foods.

We look to the opposite qualities: heat, movement, dry, light, sharp and moderation. These will assist in shedding the heavy coat of winter while we encourage the body to release stored toxins and move toward greater wellbeing.

We seek out morning hot water with lemon and ginger, or herbal chai tea, in order to stoke our digestive fire. A touch of honey can help draw excess kapha from the body. We lighten our meals from winter's comfort food. We begin to wake earlier and perform morning sun salutations or dry brushing to stimulate circulation.

We ease ourselves from hibernation and begin to shed our winter coat.

- ৪১   Exercise intensity may increase in order to provide heat and movement.

- ৪১   Add uplifting music and laughter yoga.

- ৪১   Warming stones for kapha are cat's eye and garnet.

- ৪১   Kapha benefits from essential oils that are uplifting and invigorating: eucalyptus, sweet orange, clove and cedarwood.

- ৪১   A rosemary hydrosol, or rosemary water, is a simple way to energize both skin and mind on a heavy day. Keep your hydrosol in the fridge and spray often. Close your eyes and spritz over your face, inhaling the delicate aromatherapy. Or spray your entire body and hair after a shower or bath.

- ৪১   Avoid exposure to cold and damp conditions. Seek warmth, light and movement.

৪১ SUMMER

ALTHOUGH SPRING AND fall are the recommended seasons for detoxification, there is no rule against enjoying a delicious detox during summer.

Summer may be the most naturally encouraging time to cleanse the body, particularly in a colder climate.

Summer inspires us to move our bodies, to soak in natural springs and lakes, and meditate on a star-filled sky. Summer bursts with color, making nature a natural mood booster. Increased hours of daylight offer a generous window of time in which to indulge in nourishing morning and evening practices.

Fresh produce is plentiful. Gorge on blueberries and sweet strawberries. Pick lemon balm leaves straight from your garden, and enjoy herb-infused water all day long.

Devour juicy cucumbers, sugar snap peas and succulent melons. Add bright, bountiful blackberries and raspberries to salads. Toss in fresh mint and dress with a squeeze of lemon or orange.

Sip sweet berry smoothies like lemonberry longevity tonic:

In the evening, fill ⅓ of a mason jar with dried lemon balm, then fill the remainder of the jar with hot water. Loosely cap the jar and let it sit overnight. In the morning, toss 1 cup of fresh blueberries into the blender and strain 1 cup of the lemon balm infusion over top. Add a squeeze of lemon and a touch of honey if you wish, then blend. Enjoy immediately (unless you fancy blueberry jam). If you use frozen blueberries, steep your herbs for 15-20 minutes in the morning and add the hot tea to your frozen berries before blending. Makes a brilliant breakfast. Enjoy daily.

DETOXIFICATION WITH SITALI BREATHING

ONE OF THE key channels of detoxification is the breath. It is always with us and doesn't cost a thing. *Sitali* breathing, Sanskrit for cooling or soothing, is a beneficial breathing practice for summer. If you feel overheated in the body. or find you have an overly sharp tongue or temper this summer, befriend Sitali breathing; you'll have found a cool friend indeed. Practice this breathing exercise and feel a cooler body and head prevail this season:

Sitting comfortably, extend the tongue out from the mouth.

Roll the sides of the tongue by curling the edges upward like a taco shape.

With this taco-tongue extended, draw a long, slow inhalation deep, down into the belly, like sipping through a straw.

Pull the tongue back into the mouth and exhale through the nose, long and slow, drawing the belly back toward the spine to empty the breath.

Extend the taco-tongue and take another slow, complete inhalation. No straining. Relax the belly.

Exhale again through the nose, drawing the tongue back into the mouth.

The air drawn in should feel cool while the air exiting through the nose releases heat from the body.

Continue this breathing, allowing the inhalations and exhalations to gradually lengthen as you relax and begin to cool down. Closing the eyes will assist with the calming and cooling process.

If you cannot roll up the sides of your tongue:

> Make a small *o* shape with your mouth.

> Allow your tongue to float in the middle of your mouth, not touching teeth or gums.

> Draw a long slow breath through the o-shaped lips and into the belly.

> Press the tip of the tongue against the roof of the mouth and exhale through the nose.

Sitali breathing can be done anywhere; however, it is safest to do while seated. Use this breathing practice to pacify pitta conditions: excess heat, including hot flashes in menopause, anger and agitation.

Caution should be used if you are pregnant or have low blood pressure. Discontinue if dizziness occurs.

ADDITIONAL SUGGESTIONS FOR SUMMER:

- ಠ Exercise in early morning or evening, avoiding the heat of the sun.

- ಠ Cooling stones for pitta are pearl and moonstone.

- ಠ Pitta benefits from essential oils that are both cooling and sweet: mint, jasmine, lavender and sandalwood.

- ಠ A rose hydrosol, or rosewater, is a simple and luxurious way to soothe both skin and mind on a hot day. Keep your hydrosol in the fridge and spray often. Close your eyes and spritz over your face, inhaling the delicate aromatherapy. Or spray your entire body after a shower or bath.

- ಠ Coconut water is cooling for pitta and hydrating for summer. Make a coconut water/cucumber/mint tonic in the blender, and sip in the shade.

FALL IS THE other key season for detox. This is the time of year when we prepare the body for winter. Fall is the season of vata, queen of the doshas. Her elements are air and ether; her properties are dry, light, mobile and cool. Fall's coolness may feel welcome for pitta people and the mobility from fall's winds provide movement for kapha; however, a dry and windy fall may also find monkey mind on the rise.

Scattered thoughts, increased mental chatter, restless sleep, and dry skin and nasal passages give vata's increased presence away.

Grounding, wet and warming practices may assist in bringing you back down to Earth if you feel blown away by fall.

Self-massage with oils of sesame or sweet almond infused with warming spices like cinnamon, ginger, clove, or a chai blend.

Soups and stews, roast veggie medley with carrots, onion, beets, and sweet potato or squash, all make nourishing meals for fall. Basil, ginger, and sage, or cinnamon and cardamom are warming additions to your dishes.

ADDITIONAL SUGGESTIONS FOR FALL:

- ৪ɔ Exercise in a smooth, steady way, generating warmth but not heat.

- ৪ɔ Calming and warming stones for vata are garnet and rose quartz.

- ৪ɔ Vata benefits from essential oils that are both earthy and warming: rose geranium, basil and vanilla

ഌ   A geranium hydrosol, or vanilla bean-infused water, is a
     simple and hydrating way to ease both skin and mind on a
     windy fall day. Keep your hydrosol in the fridge and spray
     often. Close your eyes and spritz over your face, inhaling
     the delicate aromatherapy. Or spray your entire body after
     a shower or bath.

ഌ   Vata benefits from an earlier bedtime and sufficient rest, as
     well as the addition of quality fats such as avocado, olive oil
     and coconut milk/oil, to meals. Avoid rough, dry food such
     as popcorn and crackers.

Take time to meditate each day, stilling the body and mind. Focus
on one task at a time, get plenty of rest, stick to a routine, and keep
life simple as you transition with the seasons and flourish this fall.

WINTER IS THE season of kapha: earth and water. The seat of kapha is the lungs. Excess kapha can present itself as congestion, lethargy, oily skin and slow digestion. Winter, however, is also a time of rest and recovery. In this season, we must strike a balance between allowing ourselves the rest and practices needed to restore ourselves, and the overindulgence of too much sleep, food and inactivity.

Those with a predominantly pitta constitution, may have little complaint when it comes to winter. You might find them buying snowshoes or cross-country skis. Kapha-dominant friends will have cozied themselves into blankets on the couch in front of a good movie. It would be wise for these friends to assist one another with balance. Kapha could benefit from joining pitta on an invigorating outdoor adventure (as long as pitta doesn't push kapha too hard), and pitta will profit from joining her friend kapha on the couch for some rest (though she'll probably fidget).

We don't generally detox during this season. We encourage and allow the body to rest and restore itself as nature does during this darker, colder time of year. This is the time for introspection and reflection.

However, this is also the season of holiday festivities and good cheer. Hence, the jump in sales of gym memberships come January, which, inevitably drop by Valentine's Day. To counter any overindulgence during December, I have created the 3-day reset in order to guide you back into balance and save you the cost of an unused gym membership.

You will find the 3-day Reset on page 47

Whether you are ready to dive deeply into the science and art that is Ayurveda, or you simply soaked up the self-care practices and seasonal suggestions, I sincerely hope you have enjoyed your Ayurveda-inspired 21-day detox.

Please remember to always be gentle with yourself and those around you. Laugh daily. Take things a little less seriously. Play beautiful music. Dance often. Spend time with family and friends. And please, practice self-care and self-love.

Thank you for participating in the detox program. It is an honor to walk with you in this life. I will see you in the Facebook group.

I leave you with one more practice.

METTA BHAVANA IS the Buddhist practice of loving kindness. This is a powerful practice for healing, forgiveness and self-love.

For more on the practice of loving kindness, visit Sharon Salzberg at www.sharonsalzberg.com.

When you recite this blessing, feel your wishes with your whole heart. Smile with your entire body as you close your eyes and see before you, in your mind's eye, yourself.

Offer yourself this blessing:

> *May I be happy*
>
> *May I be healthy*
>
> *May I be safe*
>
> *May I live with ease and joy*

You may repeat this three times (or as many times as you feel it is needed).

Then call to mind a friend or loved one. Again, smile with your whole body and offer the blessing:

> *May you be happy*
>
> *May you be healthy*
>
> *May you be safe*
>
> *May you live with ease and joy*

Feel the words as you offer them freely.

Now, call to mind an acquaintance or someone you know casually. Offer the blessing:

May you be happy

May you be healthy

May you be safe

May you live with ease and joy

Keeping the loving feeling in your heart and cells, bring to mind someone with whom you struggle. (It may take more effort to smile with your whole body here, but keep thinking good thoughts and remembering happy times).

Offer the blessing:

May you be happy

May you be healthy

May you be safe

May you live with ease and joy

Repeat several times.

Complete the practice by seeing everyone – animals, plants, rivers and oceans – as one being, and offer the blessing with great love, as I do to you now.

May you be happy

May you be healthy

May you be safe

May you be nourished

And may all beings benefit.

Namasté

ALSO BY
STEPHANIE HREHIRCHUK

Anna and the Earth Angel

Anna and the Tree Fort

AVAILABLE AT

Amazon.com

Chapters.Indigo.ca

Amazon.co.uk

Barnes & Noble

MEET THE AUTHOR

Stephanie Hrehirchuk

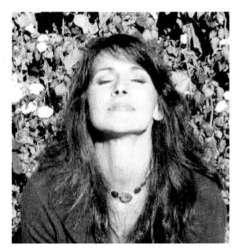

KNOWN TO RAID her grandparents' garden as a child, Stephanie has a life-long love of local food and vibrant nutrition. She has over 15 years of experience in personal training, nutrition, and wellness. Stephanie moved from working with clients in the weight room to facilitating workshops, retreats, seasonal detox programs and meditation groups. Stephanie's training includes Tibetan Breathing and Movement Yoga, meditation, raw nutrition, spinal reflexology, Qigong, Reiki, Ayurveda, plant medicine, and sustainability.

Stephanie lives in Calgary, Alberta with her husband and two children. She is the author of *Anna and the Earth Angel,* and *Anna and the Tree Fort,* with art and poetry published in the collective work *Alberta Skies.* Stephanie was a regular contributor at Gaiam, with articles published at *Sivana Spirit, Finer Minds, Guided Synergy Magazine,* and *Trifecta.* Stephanie specializes in women's issues. She writes and speaks about nutrition, health, yoga, meditation, the chakra system, parenting/motherhood, and spiritual pursuits. Stephanie has a tree planted in Alberta for every print copy sold of the Anna series of early reader books.